UNDER 500 CALORIES

THE LIGHT, QUICK

RECIPES FOR

Contents

THE SEASON AND UNDER 500 DIET

Even several centuries ago oriental philosophers and doctors noticed that different products have a different impact on the human body depending on the season. As a result of centuries-old observations and studies oriental dieticians discovered that every season activates certain organs and systems in the human body. Therefore, in order to make your body function properly and remain healthy, it is important to add certain products to your daily menu depending on the season.

Winter

The most active organ throughout the winter season is our kidneys, the main function of which is to provide proper water exchange in our body. Therefore, during the winter months it is very important to take care of the kidneys and choose the products that will promote proper nutrition for the kidneys.

In order to function well and remain healthy our kidneys need salt, which means that your daily menu should consist of meals with sufficient amount of this element. However the main secret here is to choose the proper type of salt that will be beneficial not only for kidneys, but also for the entire body as a whole. Dieticians recommend choosing large and crystallized salt with the shade of yellow. It is also possible to replace salt with natural salty products, such as soy sauce for example.

Dieticians also recommend adding more high-fat, and energy – dense products and various types of meat, such as pork, bacon and brisket, for example, especially served hot. Together with meat it is recommended to eat such side products as beans, peas, lentils and potatoes.

As it has been mentioned above, in winter salty taste is the main one, while the additional one is spicy. Therefore, feel free to add to your daily menu such products as chilli, garlic and ginger, as well as the meat of wild animals – dear, bear or moose.

Among the forbidden products in winter you will find sugar, since it suppresses the functions of the kidneys. Thus, you should avoid sweets, cakes and sweet flour products. Also, as the oriental classification states, it is better not to include to your daily ration milk and beef because they have a sweet taste.

Spring

The most active organs during the spring time are liver and gallbladder that need products with a sour taste for proper functioning. Therefore, it will be good to cook various sour soups and eat sour vegetables and fruit. It is allowed also to eat different dairy products, including cheese, milk and cottage cheese.

For meat dishes it is recommended to choose chicken, duck and turkey. It is also very important to eat beef, pork and chicken liver because exactly this meat by-product contains all the necessary microelements, the lack of which most of us feel in spring.

In the middle of spring many dieticians recommend to focus on vegetarianism that is based on the variety of vegetables, fruit and fish.

In addition to the sour taste, our liver also needs salt. Therefore, it is possible to say that in spring you are allowed to eat almost all the winter products but in reduced quantities. With regards to bitter and sweet food, it is better to either exclude it altogether or consume such products in limited quantities.

Since the liver and gallbladder are very sensitive to spicy food, it is better not to include to your menu spicy sauces and vegetables, as well as onions, garlic and the meat of wild animals.

Summer

The circulatory system, heart and small intestine are dominant parts of the human body in the summer. They are stimulated by food with a bitter taste that should play primary role in your menu. Therefore, it is good to cook salads with bitter greens and eat bitter meat, including lamb and such meat by-product as heart. It is especially good to cook meat dishes with the addition of mustard and horseradish.

Summer is the time of fresh vegetables. Among bitter vegetables choose radish, onion, cabbage, cucumbers, tomatoes, and beetroot. Pumpkins and zucchini are also good and can be used for cooking different vegetarian dishes, including pancakes, soups, porridge, and others.

Dry fruits are also believed to be good summer choices. You can either eat sweet plums, dried apples and dried apricots or make juices or desserts from them.

Sour taste is the additional one in the summer period. It is also allowed to eat some spicy and sweet food. Dieticians recommend excluding pork and beans because they are considered to be too heavy for our stomach.

By choosing drinks in summer, do not forget about the bitter taste and feel free to drink beer. However, avoid eating typical salty beer snacks, such as chips, nuts and dried fish. Instead, it is better to cook seafood and particularly shrimps.

Autumn

During this period of time there is a big strain placed on such organs as the lungs and the colon. In order to maintain them healthy and help function properly you should include spicy food to your diet. Therefore, it is recommended to use such spicy seasoning as garlic and horseradish. For the meat lovers it is recommended to choose the meat of wild animals including moose, deer, bear and wild boar. The most appropriate and healthy meat by-product in this season is lungs and liver. As a side dish it is better to choose cereals and particularly rice.

The additional autumn taste is sweet, so it is good to eat fruit and beef and also drink goat milk. As opposite, the bitter taste is forbidden, so it is not recommended to eat bitter products that might have a negative impact on your colon and the lungs. Also try to reduce the consumption of sunflower seeds and wheat flour pastry.

HOW TO COUNT CALORIES

If you keep reading this book, it means that you have already understood how important it is to count calories and to eat not more than 500 calories per serving. So, one of your main questions might be: how to count calories? Here are some useful tips on how to do it correctly and effectively in order to achieve the best results.

- ***Don't trust your memory completely.***

Even if you have an excellent memory, it is difficult to remember everything that you eat during the day. Even if you are still able to recall what you have eaten exactly, it is definitely impossible to say how much exactly you have consumed. Therefore, feel free to help yourself by keeping a special food journal or by installing a special app on your smartphone and start recording all products that reach your mouth during the day.

- ***Buy a kitchen scale***

A kitchen scale is a very useful tool that you need to have and use if you want to count calories with great precision. You do not need to weigh your meal every time, but each time when you try a new recipe, weigh a dish in order to know exactly how much you would be eating.

- ***Don't forget to count small snacks***

One of the most common mistakes the majority of people make is ignoring the small snacks. You might think that a small cereal bar that you might eat during the small break at work does not have a big influence on your daily calorie intake. However, in reality one cereal bar might contain between 100 and 150 calories. For this reason do not forget about these small snacks when you record and count calories, even if you got just a small bite.

- ***Don't ignore the major nutrients***

It is not enough to count only calories.   Pay attention to the other nutrients including fat, protein, carbohydrates and fiber because each of them is important for your overall health. For example, by increasing the fiber intake you decrease the level of trans fat, which improves your wellbeing and overall health.

APPETIZERS

- Green Frittata Muffins

- Spring Onion Pancakes

- Potato cakes

- Star and Heart pizzas

- Oat, Tomato, and Cheese Muffins

- Carrot, Hummus and Ham Mini Rolls

Green Frittata Muffins

You can be assured that the your entire family will love these healthy and delicious muffins packed with spinach, courgette, Cheddar cheese, and peas.

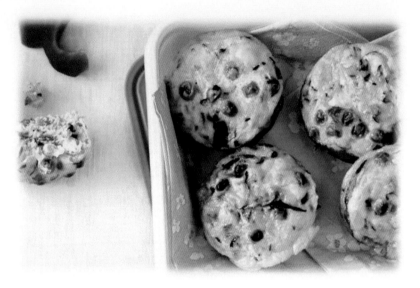

Time to cook: 30 mins

Serves: 3 (6 muffins)

Nutritional value (per serving):

115 kcal (fat – 9g, carbohydrate – 0.9g, protein – 8g , fiber – 0.4g)

Ingredients:

- Olive oil – 2 tsp
- Garlic – 1 clove
- 1/2 grated courgette
- Chopped baby spinach
- Frozen peas – 30g
- 4 beaten eggs
- Grated Cheddar cheese – 30g

Directions: First you need to grease 6 tins of a muffin tin and place a piece of baking paper inside each of them. The next step is to heat the pan with some olive oil and add the spinach, garlic and courgette. You need to cook the vegetables for 5 minutes by stirring them frequently. After this remove the pan from the heat and stir in the frozen peas. Now use a large bowl in order to mix the cooked vegetables, cheese and beaten eggs. The last step is to heat the oven (the temperature should be set at 180C) and bake your muffins for 20 minutes.

Spring Onion Pancakes

Light, fresh, healthy and easy to make pancakes can become your favourite appetizer, snack or even an entire meal.

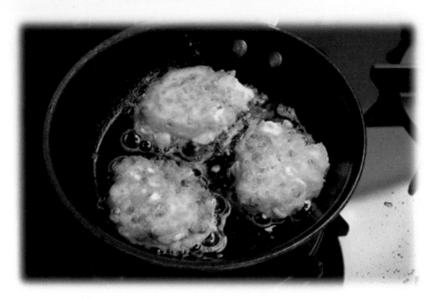

Time to cook: 25 mins

Serves: 4

Nutritional value (per serving):

210 kcal (fat – 11 , carbohydrate – 24.8g , protein – 3g , fiber – 1.6g)

Ingredients:

- Flour – 100g
- Rice flour – 25g
- 5 cut spring onions
- Freshly grounded black pepper
- Vegetable or olive oil – for frying

Directions: The first and the main step in cooking these pancakes is to combine cold water and flour. You need to add around 200ml of water a little at a time by mixing until you receive thin pancake batter. Then you need to add a pinch of black pepper and spring onions and mix thoroughly. Then turn the heat of your stove to medium-high and start frying the pancakes by forming the flat circles. Fry until golden brown on each side. Serve the pancakes with some sour cream.

Tip: Always use only cold water to make good batter and delicious pancakes.

Potato cakes

Filling and healthy potato cakes that are so easy to cook is a perfect meal for your lunch or dinner. You can combine it with pasta, porridge or any salad.

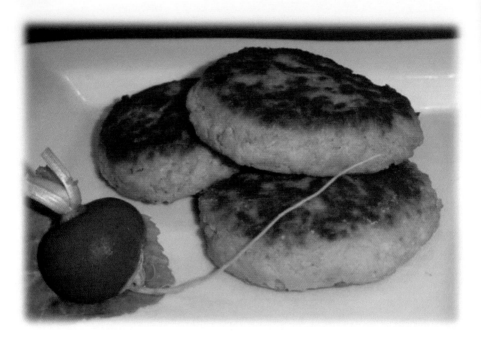

Time to cook: 1 hour

Serves: 6

Nutritional value (per serving):

124 kcal (fat – 5 , carbohydrate – 16g , protein – 2g , fiber – 0g)

Ingredients:

- 4 apples
- Potato – 1 kilo
- Flour – 4 tsp
- Horseradish – 2 tsp
- Black pepper powder – to taste
- Oil – 100 ml
- Salt – to taste

Directions: Peel the potatoes, grate them using a grater and remove the liquid by squeezing. Then do the same with the apples. After mixing the potatoes with apples, add the horseradish and the spices. Don't forget to mix everything to make homogeneous. Form oval cakes, roll them in the flour and fry until golden brown. Alternatively, to make your cakes healthier, you can bake them in the oven at 200C for 20 minutes.

Star and Heart pizzas

If you want to treat yourself or your family with something easy and delicious, then this recipe of small pizzas is perfect for you. Just 15 minutes and you will get a delicious and unusual dish full of flavours and healthy ingredients.

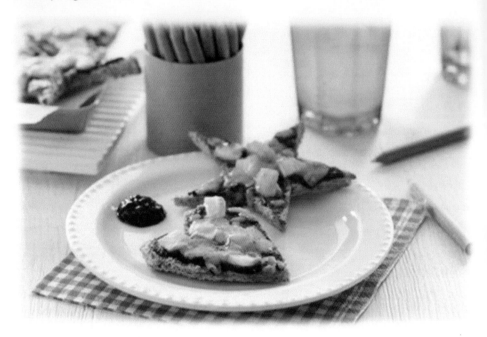

Time to cook: 15 mins

Serves: 4

Nutritional value (per serving):

173 kcal (fat – 5 , carbohydrate – 24g , protein – 9g , fibre – 4g)

Ingredients:

- Wholemeal bread – 240g (or 6 slices)
- Spray oil
- Goodness pasta sauce – 50g
- Goodness pizza flavoured cheese slices – 50g (can be replaced with grated cheddar)
- Small pineapple slices or cubes – 35g

Directions: Start with preheating the oven to 180C. The next step is rolling over the wholemeal bread or making it flat. Then cut the bread into stars or hearts, using a sharp knife or pancake moulds and place the figures on a baking sheet. You need to bake the bread for around 5 minutes until the slices become golden. Then you should spread the tomato sauce on the bread, add the cheese and top with pineapple slices. After this bake the pizzas for another 5 minutes and serve the meal hot.

Oat, Tomato, and Cheese Muffins

A very simple and delicious recipe of oat muffins that the entire family can enjoy as a snack or appetizer.

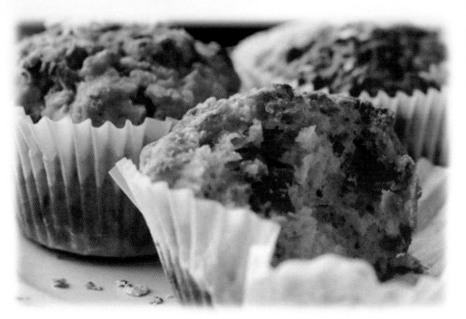

Time to cook: 30 mins

Serves: 12

Nutritional value (per serving):

190 kcal (fat – 8.7 , carbohydrate – 23g , protein – 5g , fibre – 1.6g)

Ingredients:

- Jumbo or regular rolled oats – 50g (plus 1 tbsp extra for sprinking)
- Self-rising flour – 250g
- Grated hard cheese (such as Cheddar) – 100g
- Chopped sun-dried tomatoes – 75g
- One beaten medium egg
- Melted butter – 50g
- Semi-skimmed milk – 225ml

Directions: First you need to preheat your oven to 200C, and to prepare a muffin tin with 12 holes and lined with baking papers. Then you should mix the flour, cheese and 50g of oats together. After this add tomatoes, an egg, milk and butter. Then add flour and keep mixing until you receive a batter. Put the batter in 12 holes on the muffin tin, sprinkle with 1 tbsp of oats and bake them for around 20 minutes until they become crispy and golden.

Tip: If you want some extra flavour, you can add 1 tsp of pesto sauce to the batter.

Carrot, Hummus and Ham Mini Rolls

We recommend you this tasty and healthy snack if you do not have time to cook or you are welcoming surprise guests in your house.

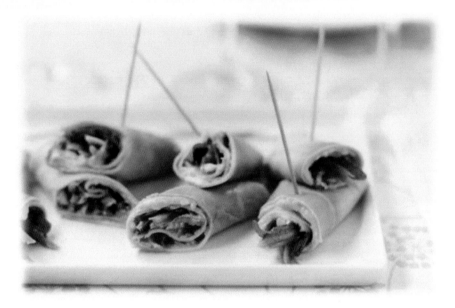

Time to cook: 5 mins

Serves: 4

Nutritional value (per serving):

28 kcal (fat – 1.1g , carbohydrate – 3.1g , protein – 1g , fibre – 1g)

Ingredients:

- Grated carrots – 50g
- Fresh orange juice – 50ml
- Hummus – 1 tbsp
- Lean ham – 4 slices
- Rocket leaves – 1 large handful
- Black pepper and salt – to taste

Directions: Mix thoroughly rocket leaves, carrots, orange juice, black pepper and salt. Add a teaspoon of this mix together with hummus to each slice of ham, wrap them around like if making rolls and secure with a toothpick.

SALADS

- The Salad with Shrimps, Arugula and Tomatoes

- Tuna and Pasta Salad

- Warm Red Pepper and Broccoli Salad

- Warm Potato and Bacon Salad

The Salad with Shrimps, Arugula and Tomatoes

The recipe of this fresh light salad is originally from the Mediterranean, where it is a popular meal for lunch or dinner. It is not only low in calories, but also very balanced, healthy and easy to cook.

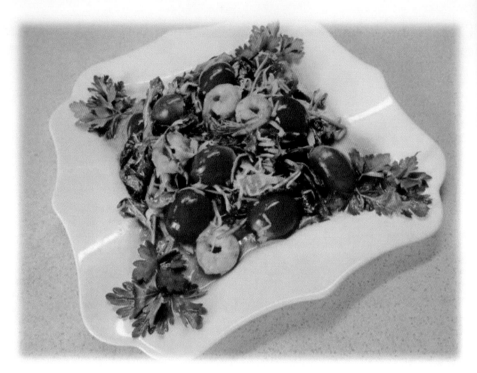

Time to cook: 10 mins

Serves: 2

Nutritional value (per serving):

97 kcal (fat – 6g , carbohydrate – 4g , protein – 6g , fiber – 0g)

Ingredients:

- Shrimps – 80g
- Hard cheese – 50g
- Cherry tomatoes – 100g
- Arugula – 150g
- Garlic – 1 clove
- Olive oil – 10ml
- Soy sauce – 10ml
- Lemon juice – 2 tsp
- Honey – 0.5 tsp
- Sea salt – to taste

Directions: You don't need any specific culinary talents in order to make this salad because it's very easy to cook. The first step is to cut garlic and fry it in a small amount of olive oil for a couple of minutes until golden brown. Then fry the shrimps for a couple of minutes from each side until they have a golden crust. After that, prepare the dressing for your salad by mixing soy sauce, honey, lemon juice, paprika powder and some oil from the pan. If you feel that it's not salty enough, feel free to add some sea salt. What remains is to cut the arugula and tomatoes, mix them with garlic and shrimps and add the dressing. If you prefer richer taste and flavour, top your culinary masterpiece with grated cheese.

Tuna and Pasta Salad

It is a classic, comfort and filling tuna salad that is very easy and quick to cook. It can become a perfect choice either for lunch or a light dinner.

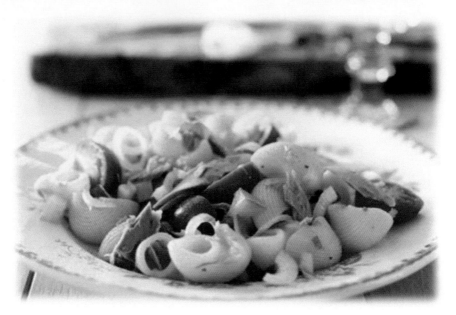

Time to cook: 30 mins

Serves: 4

Nutritional value (per serving):

445 kcal (fat – 19g , carbohydrate – 48g , protein – 23g , fiber – 2g)

Ingredients:

- Lumache – 300g
- Virgin olive oil – 50ml
- Drained and flaked canned tuna – 225g
- Halved cherry tomatoes – 100g
- 1 deseeded and finely diced green pepper
- 4 finely sliced white onions
- Salt and pepper – to taste

Directions: Start by cooking pasta that needs to be boiled in a large saucepan for 8-10 mins until al dente. When it is ready, drain and run under cold water for a couple of minutes. The last step is to put the pasta in another bowl, add the remaining ingredients from the list and mix them thoroughly. Serve the meal immediately.

Warm Red Pepper and Broccoli Salad

Despite its simplicity and easiness in preparing, this salad is laden with minerals, microelements and vitamins. Being low in calories, it is perfect for those who are eager to lose some weight. It fits well for both lunch and even late dinner.

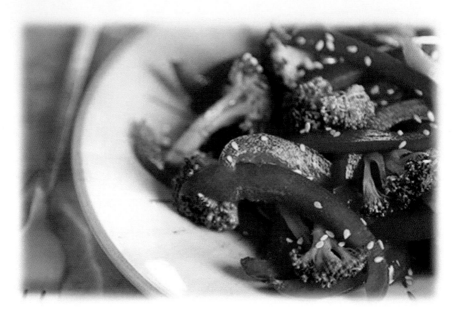

Time to cook: 25 mins

Serves: 4

Nutritional value (per serving):

96 kcal (fat – 6.5g , carbohydrate – 7g , protein – 2.6g , fiber –2.7g)

Ingredients:

- Sesame oil – 2 tbsp
- 2 finely sliced red peppers
- Broccoli – 125g
- Garlic – 1 clove
- Soy sauce – 2 tbsp
- Chilli sauce – 1.5 tsp
- Honey – 1 tsp
- Grated root ginger – 1.5 tsp
- Sesame seeds – 1 tsp

Directions: Start by heating some oil in a wok or a frying pan, after which add the sliced broccoli and peppers. It is recommended to fry the vegetables for around 5 minutes until they become golden and slightly soft. Then you need to add the remaining ingredients apart from the remaining oil and sesame seeds and stir-fry for 2-3 minutes. When the meal is ready, place it into a serving bowl or a plate and serve with some sesame seeds on top.

Warm Potato and Bacon Salad

Warm salads are a perfect way to eat healthy and add the necessary nutrients and vitamins to your daily diet. This salad with a combination of easy and affordable ingredients is a great healthy option for your lunch or dinner.

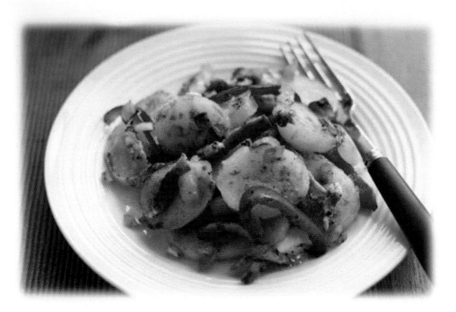

Time to cook: 30 mins

Serves: 4

Nutritional value (per serving):

234 kcal (fat – 8g , carbohydrate –33g , protein – 8g , fiber –4g)

Ingredients:

- Potatoes – 650g
- Vegetable oil – 1 tbsp
- 1 green and red diced pepper
- 1 peeled and diced onion
- 4 rashers back bacon
- Salad dressing – 1 tbsp

Directions: Cooking potatoes is the first step: you need to peel them, chop and then boil until the potatoes become tender. Meanwhile, heat the vegetable oil in a pan and cook the onion, pepper and bacon together until the onion becomes golden and soft. Add the cooked potatoes to the vegetables in the pan and toss well with the salad dressing.

SOUPS

- Chicken soup

- Onion soup

- Lentil and Chicken Soup from Morocco

- Minestrone Soup with Green Pesto

Chicken soup

Opt for this chicken soup if you want to warm your body and stomach with something comforting, delicious and healthy at the same time.

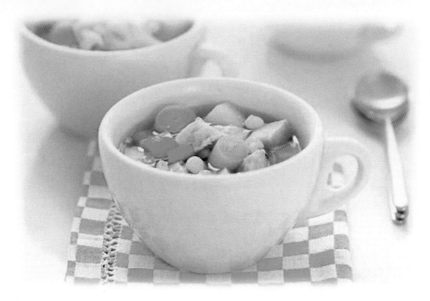

Time to cook: 50 mins

Serves: 4

Nutritional value (per serving):

198 kcal (fat – 5g , carbohydrate – 17g , protein – 18.5g , fibre – 3g)

Ingredients:

- Olive oil – 1 tbsp
- 1 diced onion
- Garlic – 1 clove
- 2 diced chicken breasts
- 2 chopped leeks
- Peeled and chopped potatoes – 200g
- Chicken stock – 1.2 litres
- Thyme – 3 sprigs
- 2 bay leaves
- Kernels from a sweet corn
- Ground black pepper – to taste

Directions: Heat the olive oil in a pan and add in the chicken, onion, garlic and leeks. Fry for around 8 minutes, making sure the meat is not becoming brown by stirring constantly. The next step is to add potatoes, thyme, chicken stock and bay leaves, and simmer for 20 minutes. The last ingredients that should be added are the kernels from a sweet corn. After 10 minutes, when the soup is ready to serve, remove the bay leaves and thyme and add some black pepper.

Onion soup

If you are a fan of soups and look for an effective recipe of the first course for your lunch or dinner, pay attention to this delicious onion soup that might become your perfect daily meal.

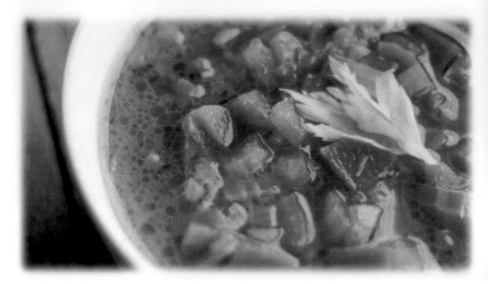

Time to cook: 1 hour

Serves: 6

Nutritional value (per serving):

32 kcal (fat – 0g , carbohydrate – 8g , protein – 2g , fibre – 0g)

Ingredients:

- Onion – 6 bulbs
- Cabbage – 1 head
- 2 carrots
- 3-4 tomatoes
- Parsley – to taste
- Spices – to taste

Directions: Chop all the vegetables into small pieces, put them into a pan and add around 5 cups of water. To make your soup more spicy and aromatic don't forget about the spices – cumin, ginger, garlic, bay leave, coriander or even some soy sauce. First you need to boil this vegetable and onion mix for 10 minutes on high heat and then continue cooking on low heat until the vegetables become soft. Serve the soup with chopped parsley on top.

Lentil and Chicken Soup from Morocco

Do you want to try something unique, international and warm in order to diversify your daily winter menu? Then you should check this aromatic Moroccan soup full of exotic flavours, lentils, vegetables and other healthy ingredients.

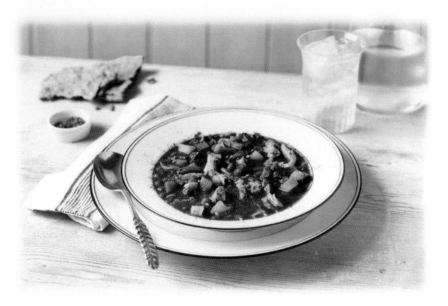

Time to cook: 45-50 mins

Serves: 4-6

Nutritional value (per serving):

173 kcal (fat – 4g , carbohydrate – 21g , protein – 15g , fiber – 5g)

Ingredients:

- Olive oil – 1 tbsp
- 1 onion
- Garlic – 2 cloves
- Cinnamon – 1 tsp
- Ground cumin – 1 tsp
- Ground coriander – 1 tsp
- Tomato puree – 2 tbsp
- Hot vegetable stock – 900 ml
- 2 carrots
- Tinned chopped tomatoes – 400g
- Tinned green lentils – 390g
- Chopped dried apricots – 100g
- 1 diced courgette
- 1 juiced and zested lemon
- Skin removed and shredded chicken breast - 245g
- Chopped fresh mint – to taste

Directions: Start by heating the oil over medium heat and frying the garlic and onion for 3-4 minutes until they become soft. Then it's time to add cumin, cinnamon, tomato puree and coriander and cook for 2-3 minutes more. The following step is to add the carrots and the stock and simmer the mixture for 6-7 minutes. When the carrots get softened, stir in the chopped dried apricots, tomatoes and lentils and simmer for 15 minutes. After that add the courgette and chicken that should be cooked for 5 minutes, after which you need to add the last ingredient - the lemon juice. To serve this soup properly, do not forget to top it with fresh mint and lemon zest.

Minestrone Soup with Green Pesto

This soup loaded with flavours and fresh vegetables is a perfect homemade and comforting meal for a cold winter day. Try this recipe and get carried away by the atmosphere of sunny Italy.

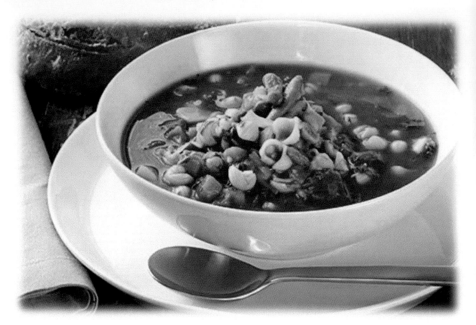

Time to cook: 20 mins

Serves: 2

Nutritional value (per serving):

184 kcal (fat – 8 , carbohydrate – 18g , protein – 12g , fibre – 7.5g)

Ingredients:

- Olive oil – 1 tsp
- 1 peeled and chopped onion
- 0.5 chopped red pepper
- 1 peeled and diced carrot
- Vegetable stock – 500 ml
- Cherry tomatoes – 400g
- Oregano – 1tsp
- Defrosted soya beans – 250g
- Green pesto – 2tsp
- Ground black pepper
- Grated parmigiano cheese - to taste and serve

Directions: Heat some olive oil in a pan with and add the onion, pepper and carrots. You should cook this mixture for around 5 minutes until vegetables become a bit tender and brown. The next step is adding the vegetable stock and then spaghetti. Reduce the heat to low and continue cooking for another 6-7 minutes. Finally, put soya beans, tomatoes and oregano and bring it back to a boil. Cook until the pasta is cooked and do not forget to stir regularly.

SIDE DISHES

- Vichy Carrots

- Asparagus with Romesco Sauce

- Rosemary Crispy Potatoes

- Cauliflower and Lentil Pilaf

- Thai Green Vegetable Curry

Vichy Carrots

Carrot is one of the healthiest vegetable that can be easily found in any supermarket, and there are many recipes of carrot dishes. We offer one of them that can easily become one of your favourite side dishes served with meat or a salad.

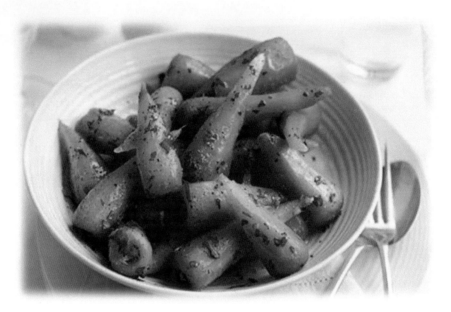

Time to cook: 30 mins

Serves: 6

Nutritional value (per serving):

61 kcal (fat – 2.7g , carbohydrate – 8.7g , protein – 1g , fiber –4g)

Ingredients:

- Chantenay carrots – 750g
- Butter – 15g
- Sugar – 2 tsp
- Honey – 2 tbsp
- Chopped fresh parsley – 2 tbsp

Directions: Halve several large carrots and put them into a saucepan and mix them with sugar, butter and a pinch of salt. The next step is covering the carrots half way with water and bringing them to a boil. Keep cooking at a simmer for another 15-20 minutes until the carrots become soft. Then you should turn up the heat to medium-high and continue cooking until you get a buttery glaze. In the end, stir in the parsley and serve.

Asparagus with Romesco Sauce

Asparagus is definitely one of those superfoods you can't avoid in your diet. Try this vegetarian and light recipe of asparagus with romesco sauce that can become a perfect addition to your lunch or dinner.

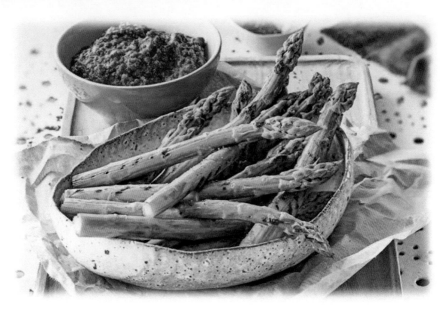

Time to cook: 20 mins

Serves: 6

Nutritional value (per serving):

198 kcal (fat – 17.4g , carbohydrate – 6g , protein – 5.3g , fiber –0.5g)

Ingredients:

- Trimmed asparagus – 500g
- Olive oil – 1 tbsp

For the sauce

- Drained jar roasted peppers – 285g
- Toasted blanched almonds – 100g
- Garlic – 1 clove
- Sherry vinegar – 1 tbsp
- Crushed red chilli flakes – 1 tsp
- Rustic white bread (torn into pieces) – 25g
- Smoked paprika – 0.5 tsp
- Tomato puree – 1 tbsp
- Virgin olive oil – 60 ml

Directions: Put the sauce ingredients into a food processor and mix them while adding the oil gradually until you receive a coarse paste. When the sauce is ready put it in a separate bowl. Then toss asparagus with oil and fry it in a griddle pan until it becomes charred (for around 3-4 minutes). Serve with the sauce you prepared before.

Rosemary Crispy Potatoes

Crispy golden potatoes are always a great choice for a side dish. This recipe is much easier than a regular one because you do not need to boil potatoes first. Instead, you just need to put them chucked into the oven together with aromatic rosemary.

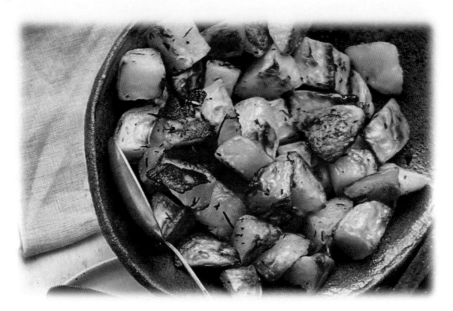

Time to cook: 40 mins

Serves: 6

Nutritional value (per serving):

113 kcal (fat – 3g , carbohydrate – 20g , protein – 2g , fiber –2g)

Ingredients:

- Chopped potatoes – 700g
- Olive oil – 1.5 tbsp
- 2 chopped springs of rosemary leaves

Directions: First of all preheat your oven to 220C. Place the chopped potatoes in a roasting tin and add some olive oil, rosemary, and some salt. After this toss everything well to coat. You need to bake the potatoes for around 30-40 minutes until they become golden and crispy.

Cauliflower and Lentil Pilaf

This delicious, aromatic and easy-to-cook meal can become a perfect and exquisite side dish for your lunch or dinner. Due to its nutritious ingredients it can be fairly called not only a filling, but also a very healthy dish.

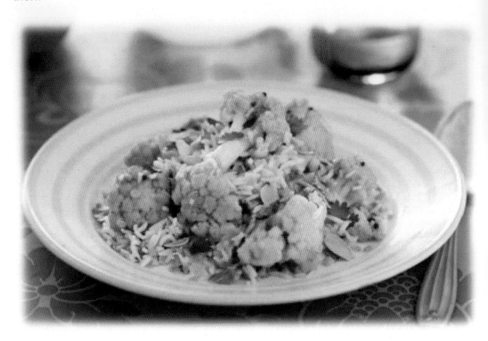

Time to cook: 45 mins

Serves: 4

Nutritional value (per serving):

330 kcal (fat – 10.7g , carbohydrate – 47g , protein – 15g , fiber –7.5g)

Ingredients:

- Basmati rice – 100g
- Red lentils - 150g
- Olive oil – 2 tbsp
- Mustard seeds – 1 tsp
- 1 peeled onion
- A half of diced red chilli
- Turmeric – 0.5 tsp
- Ground coriander – 0.5 tsp
- 1 cauliflower
- Vegetable stock – 2 tbsp
- Toasted flaked almonds – 2 tbsp
- Chopped coriander – 2 tbsp

Directions: First of all you need to cook the lentils and rice according to the instructions provided on the packs. Meanwhile, heat a pan with olive oil and fry mustard seeds until they start to pop. After this add garlic and chilli, cook them for 2-3 minutes and add the spices. One minute later stir in the cauliflower and then add the vegetable stock. This mixture should be left covered on the stove on low heat for around 5 minutes until the cauliflower becomes soft. The final step is stirring in the lentils and rice together with chopped coriander and flaked almonds.

Thai Green Vegetable Curry

Originally from Thailand, this variant of curry is a perfect and healthy choice for those, who are watching their diet. In addition, it is absolutely fragrant, delicious and quick to make.

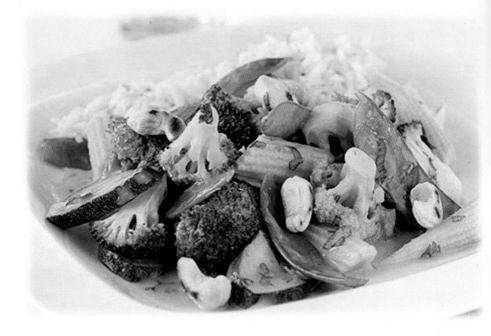

Time to cook: 25 mins

Serves: 4

Nutritional value (per serving):

223 kcal (fat – 15g , carbohydrate – 10g , protein – 10.5g , fibre –6g)

Ingredients:

- Reduced-fat coconut milk – 400ml
- Thai green curry paste – 2 tbsp
- 2 sliced courgettes of a medium size
- Broccoli – 1 head
- Snow peas or mangetouts – 150g
- Baby sweet corn – 150g
- Unsalted cashew nuts – 50g
- Ground coriander – 0.5 tsp

Directions: Mix together the coconut milk with green curry paste in a wide pan and bring to a simmer. After a couple minutes it is time to add the courgettes and cook for another 5 minutes. Divide the broccoli head into small florets and add them to the pan together with the baby corn and mangetouts. Cooking time of this mix, that should be simmered gently, is 5 minutes.

Tip: *We recommend you to serve this meal with either rice noodles or rice.*

MAIN DISHES

- Asian Salmon Fillet

- Fried Marinated Chicken

- Creamy Pasta with Mint

- Fusilli Pasta with Roasted Peppers

- Light Tuna Fishcakes

- Tuna steaks with a chilli and caper marinade

Asian Salmon Fillet

If you are a fan of seafood and want to try something a little bit exotic, then you should cook and taste the salmon fillet inspired by the flavours from Asia. The delicious taste of this dish will definitely blow you away.

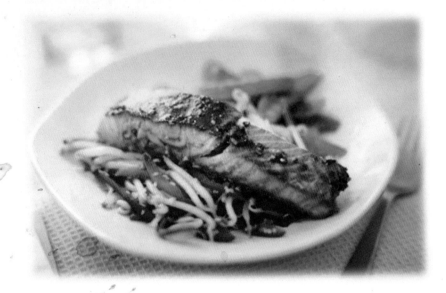

Time to cook: 30 mins

Serves: 4

Nutritional value (per serving):

342 kcal (fat – 21g , carbohydrate – 9g , protein – 27g , fiber –3g)

Ingredients:

- Salmon Fillets – 480g
- Soy sauce – 1.5 tbsp
- Caster sugar – 1 tsp
- Juice of one lime
- 2 cm piece of peeled and chopped ginger
- Garlic – 2 cloves
- Sesame oil – 1.5 tbsp
- 2 sliced red peppers
- Fresh bean sprouts – 200g
- Sesame seeds – 10g

Directions: The first step is to marinate the salmon. In order to do this you need to put the salmon fillets into a non-metallic shallow dish and add the mixture of such ingredients as sugar, soy sauce and lime juice. Then after deseeding the chilli, peeling and chopping the garlic and ginger, mix them all together and add to your fish. The salmon should be covered and left for 10 minutes for marinating better.

Meanwhile heat a pan and fry the red peppers in some oil for a couple of minutes. Add fresh the bean sprouts and fry this mixture for one more minute. After this it is time to add your salmon to the pan together with marinating juices and fry it covered for about 10 minutes or until well cooked-through.

Tips: *For a better taste it is recommended to add 80g of steamed sugar snap peas, yet it adds extra 33 kcal.*

Fried Marinated Chicken

It is a crispy grilled and healthy alternative to a classic fried chicken that can be perfectly served with vegetables, porridge or salad.

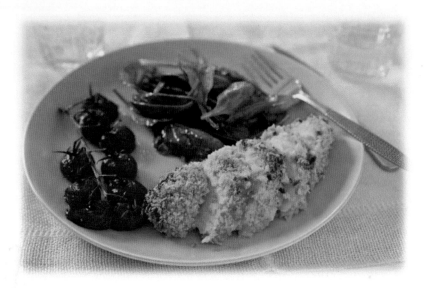

Time to cook: 40 mins

Serves: 4

Nutritional value (per serving):

298 kcal (fat – 9g , carbohydrate – 22.7g , protein – 31.5g , fiber –1g)

Ingredients:

- 4 boneless and skinless chicken breasts (alternatively you can use chicken fillets)
- Buttermilk – 284ml
- Panko breadcrumbs – 100g
- Zest of one lemon
- Grated parmesan cheese – 20g
- Olive oil – 2 tbsp

Directions: Marinating the chicken is the first step of the cooking process: you should put the breasts or fillets into a mixing bowl, add buttermilk, cover and leave it for at least 2 hours. It is even recommended to leave it overnight, so the meat would get even softer. The next step is to preheat the grill, take a deep shallow bowl and mix lemon zest, Parmesan cheese and breadcrumbs. After removing the chicken from the milk marinade, cover it with breadcrumb mix and drizzle with the olive oil. Then the meat should be grilled until it becomes golden from both sides (about 15 minutes in total).

Creamy Pasta with Mint

If you want something fresh and easy for your lunch or dinner, pay attention to this simple and unusual recipe of pasta. Easy and fast to make – it will occupy a worthy place in your recipe book.

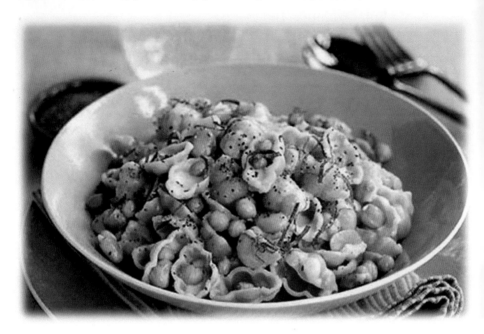

Time to cook: 25 mins

Serves: 4

Nutritional value (per serving):

478 kcal (fat – 22g , carbohydrate – 60.9 , protein – 16.8 , fibre –11g)

Ingredients:

- Wholewheat conhiglie – 400g
- Frozen peas – 145g
- Broad beans – 145g
- Creme Fraiche – 200ml
- Vegetable stock - 300ml
- Fresh mint – 30g
- Ground black pepper – to taste

Directions: First of all boil the pasta in a large pan according the instructions on the pack. When the pasta is ready, add the beans and peas and simmer this mixture for a couple of minutes. Meanwhile, put the crème fraiche and the vegetable stock into a saucepan. Then place it on the stove over low heat and leave for around 5 minutes to heat up. It is very important to stir constantly and to avoid boiling. The final step is to mix the crème fraiche sauce with pasta and vegetables and serve the dish immediately while it is hot.

Fusilli Pasta with Roasted Peppers

If you still think that pasta cannot be healthy and low-calorie, then you should definitely try this recipe of fusilli pasta with peppers – the source of energy, Italian flavours, and healthy microelements.

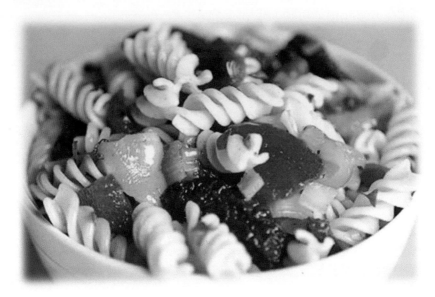

Time to cook: 50 mins

Serves: 4

Nutritional value (per serving):

432 kcal (fat – 8.4g , carbohydrate – 80.5 , protein – 12 , fibre –9g)

Ingredients:

- 1 large red and 1 yellow pepper
- Olive oil – 1 tbsp
- 2 chopped shallots
- Garlic – 1 clove
- Crushed dried chillies – 1 tsp
- Vegetable stock – 100ml
- Sundried, drained and chopped tomatoes – 125g
- Balsamic vinegar – 2 tbsp
- Dried fusilli pasta – 350g

Directions: First, preheat the oven. The temperature should be 230C. Put the yellow and red peppers into an ovenproof dish and bake them for a half an hour until they become softened. When cooked, leave them for 10 minutes, then remove the skin and chop them. Then take a saucepan and heat the oil in it, then add the shallots and cook them until soft. The following ingredients to add are garlic, vegetable stock and chillies that you need to cook for around 5 minutes. After this you can add tomatoes and peppers together with the rest of the stock and leave this mixture to simmer for another 10 minutes. At the end pour some vinegar. The final step is to add the cooked fusilli pasta, mix all the ingredients together and serve.

Light Tuna Fishcakes

Do you want something light and easy for your lunch or dinner? Then try these fishcakes made of tuna. You can enjoy them with rice or salad.

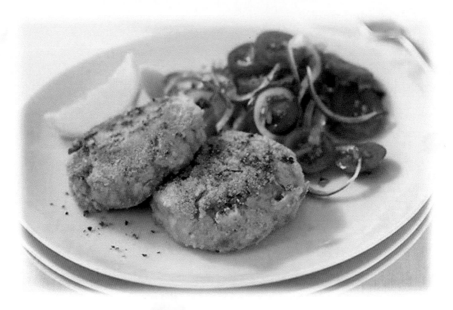

Time to cook: 45 mins

Serves: 4

Nutritional value (per serving):

408 kcal (fat – 11g , carbohydrate – 49g , protein – 24.6g , fibre –5.6g)

Ingredients:

- Peeled and chopped sweet potatoes – 600g
- Tuna in sauce – 300g
- 2 chopped spring onions
- 1 egg
- Freshly ground black pepper
- Breadcrumbs – 100g
- Olive oil – 3 tbsp
- 1 lemon – for serving

Directions: Start with cooking sweet potatoes by boiling them for 20 minutes. When the potatoes are ready, drain well and mash them. Add the tuna, egg, spring onions, black pepper and then mix them thoroughly. Divide the mixture into several parts, shape into balls, and roll them in breadcrumbs. Finally, fry them on each side for several minutes until golden. It is recommended to serve them with lemon and vegetable salad.

Tuna steaks with a chilli and caper marinade

This is a healthy and delicious recipe of original steaks that can make your lunch or dinner very special.

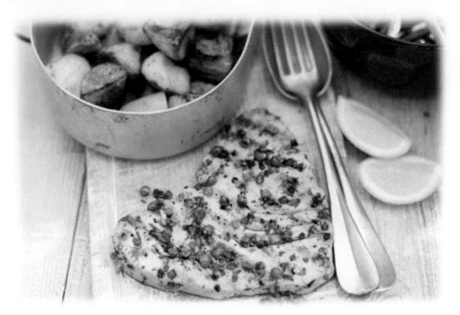

Time to cook: 15 mins

Serves: 4

Nutritional value (per serving):

224 kcal (fat – 11g , carbohydrate – 0.5g , protein – 30g , fibre –0.3g)

Ingredients:

- 1 deseeded and finely chopped red chilli
- Garlic – 1 clove
- Small capers – 1 tbsp
- Chopped parsley – 2 tbsp
- A half of a juiced lemon
- Virgin olive oil- 2 tbsp
- 4 tuna steaks
- Steamed fine green beans and crispy potatoes – for serving

Directions: Take a small bowl and mix in garlic, lemon juice, chilli and some oil. Then put the tuna steaks into the bowl and toss well with the rest of the ingredients. Leave them covered with the marinade for one hour. After this heat the barbecue and fry the steaks for several minutes each side. The cooking time will depend on how thick the steaks are. Enjoy your meal together with potatoes or green beans.

DESSERTS

- Tangerine and Melon Fruit Salad

- Mango, honey and almond smoothie

- Buttermilk Fruity Pancakes

- Ginger and Pineapple Sweet Salsa

- Fresh Berry and Banana Salad

This delicious and light fruit salad with juicy melon, pomegranates and tangerines is a healthy and simple recipe that takes not more than 10 minutes to make. Enjoy it as a healthy and fresh breakfast or a light dessert.

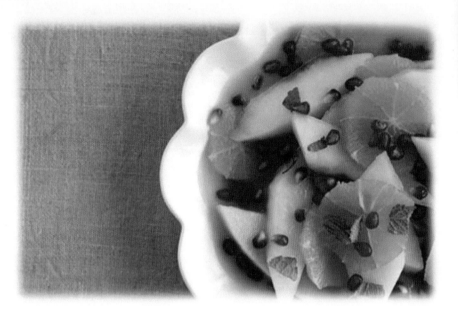

Time to cook: 10 mins

Serves: 8

Nutritional value (per serving):

90 kcal (fat – 0g , carbohydrate – 21g , protein – 2g , fibre – 4g)

Ingredients:

- 1 honeydew melon
- 4 tangerines
- Juice of 2 tangerines
- 2 pomegranates
- 2 limes

Directions: Cut the melon into quarters and do not forget to remove all the seeds. Then cut off its skin and slice into long pieces. Use a serrated knife for cutting the skin and pith of the tangerines, and then slice them. The pomegranates should also be cut into quarters and deseeded. When the fruits are ready, mix them in a large bowl by adding the juice of 2 tangerines and limes. You can add some organic honey if needed for a sweeter taste.

Mango, honey and almond smoothie

If you want to start your morning with something healthy, filling, nutritional and sweet, then this smoothie is a perfect choice. It is a great cocktail that is perfect for both adults and kids.

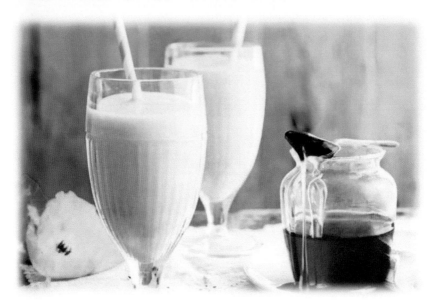

Time to cook: 5 min

Serves: 2

Nutritional value (per serving):

265 kcal (fat – 7.5g , carbohydrate – 35g , protein – 15g , fiber – 2.5g)

Ingredients:

-   1 mango
-   ½ cup of low-fat yoghurt
-   400 ml of skim milk
-   Manuka honey – 1 tbs
-   Almond meal – 2 tbs
-   Ice cubes – to taste

Directions: First peel and cut a mango into small pieces. Put it into a blender together with the skim milk, almond meal, yoghurt and manuka honey. If you want your smoothie to be cooler, also add several ice cubes. Blend all the ingredients together until smooth and divide the cocktail between two glasses.

Buttermilk Fruity Pancakes

If you lack good ideas for sweet and delicious breakfast or just want to pamper yourself with something filling and healthy, then this recipe of sweet and easy-to-cook pancakes is the real deal.

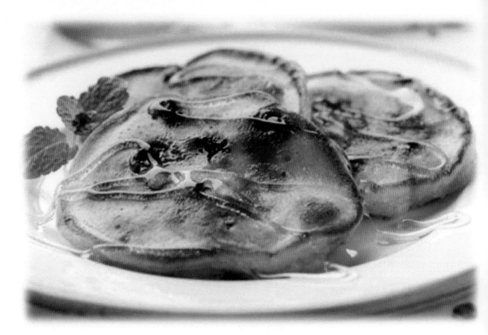

Time to cook: 15 min

Serves: 2

Nutritional value (per serving):

268 kcal (fat – 8.3g , carbohydrate – 42.8g , protein – 8g , fiber –1.8g)

Ingredients:

- Self-rising flour - 150g
- 2 medium-sized eggs
- Buttermilk – 150ml
- Honey – 2 tbsp
- Raspberries or blueberries – 100g
- Rapeseed oil – 2 tbps

Directions: Take a large bowl and add the flour. Add honey and eggs, and then whisk in the buttermilk together with rapeseed oil in order to get a thick batter. The final preparatory step is to add the berries into the dough. After heating a pan with some oil, spoon some mixture into the pan while forming four pancakes. Fry them for 2-3 minutes on each side. In total you will get 12 pancakes.

Ginger and Pineapple Sweet Salsa

A dessert should be not only sweet but also healthy. For this reason we offer you this recipe of the fresh sweet salsa with a mixture of exotic fruits and flavours.

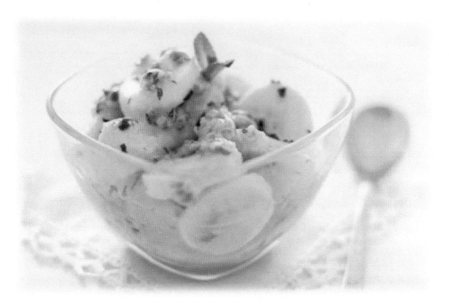

Time to cook: 5 mins

Serves: 4

Nutritional value (per serving):

90 kcal (fat – 1g , carbohydrate – 22g , protein – 1g , fibre–2.5g)

Ingredients:

- Fresh and chopped pineapple – 400g
- 3 passion fruit
- 1 chopped banana
- Fresh mint – 1 tbsp
- Peeled and grated ginger – 4 tsp
- Pineapple juice – 150 ml
- Salt – to taste

Directions: This desert is probably the easiest thing to cook. All you need to do is to mix the slices of passion fruit and pineapple, ginger and pineapple juice. At the end, add the chopped banana and a pinch of salt. Mix well all the ingredients and add some fresh mint on the top for decoration.

Fresh Berry and Banana Salad

This salad is not just very fresh and delicious, but also quite nutritional, which makes it a perfect breakfast or dessert.

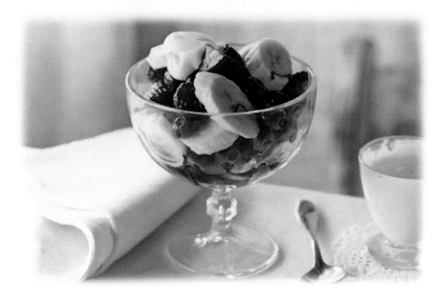

Time to cook: 15 mins

Serves: 4

Nutritional value (per serving):

159 kcal (fat – 0.5g , carbohydrate – 32g , protein – 1g , fibre–6.7g)

Ingredients:

- Juice of one orange
- Honey – 1 tbsp
- 15 shredded mint leaves
- Halved and hulled strawberries – 300g
- Blueberries – 250g
- Raspberries – 225g
- 2 peeled and sliced bananas
- Natural yogurt – for serving

Directions: Mix honey and orange juice in a small pan and heat until the honey starts melting. Then leave the syrup to cool and after add some mint leaves in it. Put all the prepared fruit slices and berries in a serving bowl and pour over the honey syrup. Finally add some natural yogurt and enjoy your fresh and sweet meal.

CONCLUSION

We truly believe that this book will help you change your perception of healthy nutrition and expand your collection of healthy, delicious and original recipes. We also hope that it can become not just another cooking book, but rather a useful guide to a healthy lifestyle and the world of a wide variety of tastes.

We are thankful for reading our book, trying our recipes and sharing our passion for healthy nutrition.

Legal & Disclaimer

The information contained in this book and its contents is not designed to replace or take the place of any form of medical or professional advice; and is not meant to replace the need for independent medical, financial, legal or other professional advice or services, as may be required. The content and information in this book has been provided for educational and entertainment purposes only.

The content and information contained in this book have been compiled from sources deemed reliable, and it is accurate to the best of the Author's knowledge, information and belief. However, the Author cannot guarantee its accuracy and validity and cannot be held liable for any errors and/or omissions. Further, changes are periodically made to this book as and when needed. Where appropriate and/or necessary, you must consult a professional (including but not limited to your doctor, attorney, financial advisor or such other professional advisor) before using any of the suggested remedies, techniques, or information in this book.

Upon using the contents and information contained in this book, you agree to hold harmless the Author from and against any damages, costs, and expenses, including any legal fees potentially resulting from the application of any of the information provided by this book. This disclaimer applies to any loss, damages or injury caused by the use and application, whether directly or indirectly, of any advice or information presented, whether for breach of contract, tort, negligence, personal injury, criminal intent, or under any other cause of action.

You agree to accept all risks of using the information presented inside this book.

You agree that by continuing to read this book, where appropriate and/or necessary, you shall consult a professional (including but not limited to your doctor, attorney, or financial advisor or such other advisor as needed) before using any of the suggested remedies, techniques, or information in this book.

- notes

Printed in Great Britain
by Amazon